SECRET RECIPES ON VEGETARIAN COOKING SPECIFIC TO THE TASTIEST FRUIT DISHES

A Recipe Book Not To Be Missed For Lovers Of Vegetarian Cooking All The Most Delicious Recipes Of Fruit That Will Allow You To Lose Weight In A Simple And Fast Way All Explained Step By Step For Beginners.

Alberto Garofano

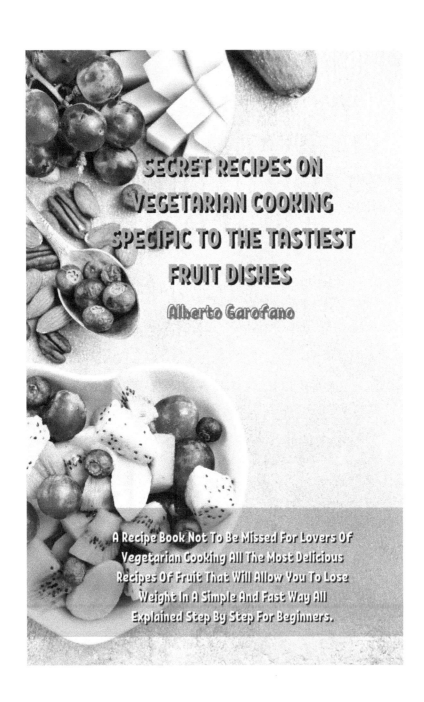

SECRET RECIPES ON VEGETARIAN COOKING SPECIFIC TO THE TASTIEST FRUIT DISHES

Alberto Garofano

A Recipe Book Not To Be Missed For Lovers Of
Vegetarian Cooking All The Most Delicious
Recipes Of Fruit That Will Allow You To Lose
Weight In A Simple And Fast Way All
Explained Step By Step For Beginners.

Table Of Contents

The information in the following pages is broadly considered a truthful and accurate account of facts and as such, any inattention, use, or misuse of the information in question by the reader will render any resulting actions solely under their purview. There are no scenarios in which the publisher or the original author of this work can be in any fashion deemed liable for any hardship or damages that may befall them after undertaking information described herein.

Additionally, the information in the following pages is intended only for informational purposes and should thus be thought of as universal. As befitting its nature, it is presented without assurance regarding its prolonged validity or interim quality. Trademarks that are mentioned are done without written consent and can in no way be considered an endorsement from the trademark holder.

☆ 55% OFF for BookStore NOW at $ 30,95 instead of $ 41,95! ☆

A Recipe Book Not To Be Missed For Lovers Of

Vegetarian Cooking All The Most Delicious

Recipes Of Fruit That Will Allow You To Lose

Weight In A Simple And Fast Way All

Explained Step By Step For Beginners.

Buy is NOW and let your Customers get addicted to this amazing book!

INTRODUCTION

The vegetarian diet in Italy is spreading widely both for the ease with which vegetables are found in the markets and because they have always been present in the Mediterranean diet. Furthermore, in recent years, with the progressive increase of the world population and the continuous exploitation of the earth's resources, feeding models are being enhanced that have a low environmental impact and can be used for a long time. From these assumptions, diets are born that partially or completely avoid foods of animal origin: the vegetarian diet that does not involve the consumption of meat and fish, molluscs and crustaceans, but allows, in different ways, the consumption of eggs. And dairy products; the vegan diet which, on the other hand, eliminates all products of animal origin.

Following the indications contained in the Guidelines for healthy eating, the vegetarian diet can be formulated to meet the needs of a healthy adult:

- Eat more portions of vegetables and fresh fruit every day
- Increase the consumption of legumes, both fresh and dried
- regularly consume bread, pasta, rice and other cereals , preferably wholemeal.
- Eat moderate amounts of fats and oils used for seasoning and cooking. Above all, limit fats of

animal origin (butter, lard, lard, cream, etc.) to season foods and prefer fats of vegetable origin: extra virgin olive oil and seed oils, preferably raw.

- Consume eggs and milk that contain good organic quality proteins. If you drink a lot of milk, preferably choose the skim or semi-skim one which, however, maintains its calcium and vitamin content.
- Eat cheeses in moderate quantities because in addition to proteins they contain high amounts of fat. For this reason it is advisable to choose the leaner ones, or eat smaller portions
- Limit foods rich in fat, salt and sugar such as creams, chocolate, chips, biscuits, sweets, ice cream, cakes and puddings to special occasions

The Elements That Cannot Be Missing In A Vegetarian Diet

The first thing to watch out for is to follow a diet that is as varied as possible. Some nutrients are present in small amounts in vegetables, or are less easily absorbed by the body than those from meat or fish. However, most vegetarians generally do not have ailments due to nutrient deficiencies if they take care to include certain foods in their diet:

- Legumes combined with cereals, to ensure the availability, in addition to significant quantities of starch and fiber, of essential nutrients characteristic of meat, fish and eggs, such as iron, proteins of good biological quality, micro nutrients

- Foods obtained from wholemeal flours (and not with the simple addition of bran or other fibers) which, in addition to starch and fiber, contain good amounts of calcium, iron and B vitamins

If not formulated correctly, the vegetarian diet can be deficient in essential nutrients. Those who follow it need to make sure they get sufficient amounts of iron and vitamin B12 with their food.

Plant Sources Of Iron

Vegetarians may have less iron in their body stores than people who also eat meat. It is therefore important to know the foods, suitable for vegetarians, which contain a good amount of iron:

- Eggs
- Legumes (especially lentils)
- Dried fruit
- Pumpkin seeds
- Vegetables (especially dark green ones)
- Whole grain bread
- Plant Sources of Vitamin B12

Vitamin B12 is needed for growth, cell repair, and overall health. It is found, in nature, only in products of animal origin such as, for example, meat, fish, shellfish, eggs and dairy products. If you eat these foods regularly, you are likely to be getting enough of them. However, if you only eat small amounts of foods of animal origin, or if you avoid them altogether, it is important to include certain sources of vitamin B12 in your diet:

- Milk
- Cheese
- Eggs

If the amount of vitamin B12 introduced in the diet is insufficient to meet the body's needs, it is advisable to also use foods in which it is added (fortified foods) such as:

- Fortified breakfast cereals
- Fortified soy products
- Plant sources of omega-3

The omega-3 fatty acids are found mainly in oily fish, fresh tuna and salmon. Plant sources of omega-3 fatty acids include:

- Flax seed
- Rapeseed oil
- Soybean oil and soy-based foods (such as tofu)
- Nuts

Being Vegetarian In Particular Conditions

Those who wish to follow a vegetarian diet during childhood, pregnancy, advanced age or in conjunction with illnesses, must rely on a doctor or nutritionist, because in such conditions their needs for nutrients may vary. For example, during pregnancy and breastfeeding, women following a vegetarian diet need to ensure that the amounts of vitamins and minerals in their diet are sufficient to ensure that their baby can grow healthily. While growing up, the parent must ensure that the child eats a very varied diet to meet the nutritional needs he needs.

START

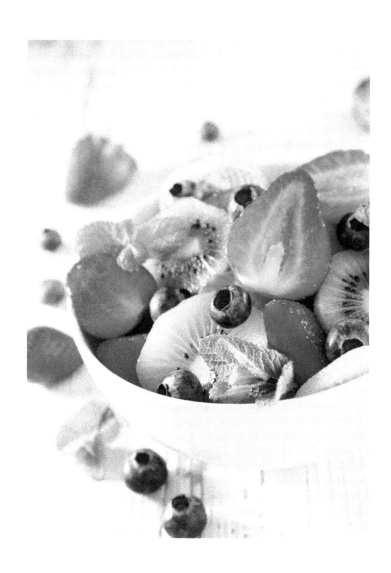

Oranges with Italian fennel salad

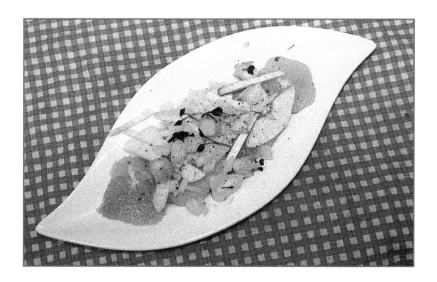

Servings:2

INGREDIENTS

- 1 thick Fennel bulb
- 1 small Onion (s), red
- 1 tbsp Red wine vinegar
- Sea salt and pepper, black
- 6 tbsp Olive oil, very good, mild
- 4th Orange
- 2 tbsp Kalamata olives, in brine, without stone

PREPARATION

Wash the fennel. Cut off the stems. Quarter the tuber and remove the stalk. Cut the fennel into very fine slices with a large knife.
Pluck the greens off the stems, chop them up and set aside.
Peel the onion, cut in half and cut into fine slices.
Put the fennel with the onions in a bowl and dress with red wine vinegar, salt, pepper and olive oil. Stir everything well and let it steep for 10 minutes.
In the meantime, peel the oranges and cut them into slices.
Arrange the orange slices on 2 large plates and place half of the fennel salad in the middle. Spread the olives on top and sprinkle with a little olive oil, fennel greens and black pepper.

Italian strawberry and mascarpone cream

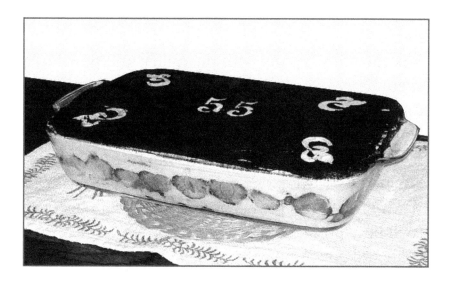

Servings:6

INGREDIENTS

- 750 g Strawberries
- 100 g powdered sugar
- 500 g Mascarpone
- 250 g Quark (low-fat quark)
- 150 g Biscuit (Amarettini)

PREPARATION

Clean and wash the strawberries, then puree 250g of them.

Mix the mascarpone with the quark and powdered sugar.

Cut the remaining strawberries into slices.

Now layer in a mold as follows: strawberries, mascarpone cream, half of the amarettini (will not be crushed), strawberry puree, mascarpone cream, strawberries and the second half of the amarettini (will be crumbled beforehand).

Chill and consume within the next 2 hours.

Strawberry curd with amaretti

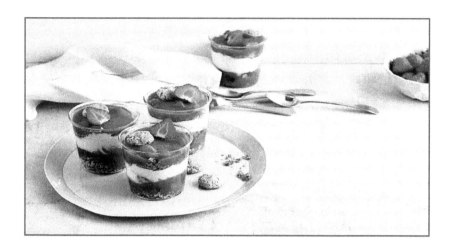

Servings:4
- 500 g Strawberries
- 500 g Quark
- 200 g sweet cream
- 2 tbsp Sugar or candarel
-

PREPARATION

Puree 300 g of the strawberries.
If the strawberries are not sweet enough, add 1
tablespoon of sugar or candarel if necessary.
Leave 4 beautiful strawberries as decoration, finely
dice the rest and add to the pureed mixture.

Beat the quark with the sugar or candarel until frothy. Whip the whipped cream until stiff, if you like, with pure vanilla or season it and carefully fold it into the quark.

Keep a few of the amaretti for decoration, coarsely grind the rest in a blender or crumble in a plastic bag with a rolling pin.

Set up 4 large, bulbous glasses, put a layer of amaretti crumbs in each glass, top with quark, then strawberry puree, then amaretti crumbs, again quark and strawberries. The last layer should be amaretti crumbs, decorate with whole amaretti and the strawberries.

Can be prepared well. Can be put in the fridge in the morning, but not overnight, please!

Crema di fragola

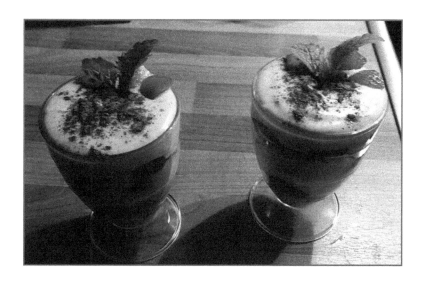

Servings:3

INGREDIENTS

- 2 Egg
- 50 g sugar
- 250 g Mascarpone
- 150 g Strawberries
- Cocoa powder
- Mint, fresh

PREPARATION

Separate the eggs and beat the egg whites until stiff.
Then beat the egg yolks with the sugar until creamy
until the sugar crystals have dissolved.
Add the mascarpone to the sugar and egg yolk
mixture and stir to form a homogeneous mixture.
Then fold this mixture into the stiff egg white.
Clean the strawberries and cut into pieces.
Spread the cream on top.
You can also layer the strawberries and cream.
Garnish with cocoa powder and a fresh mint leaf if
you like.

Pizza Chiquita

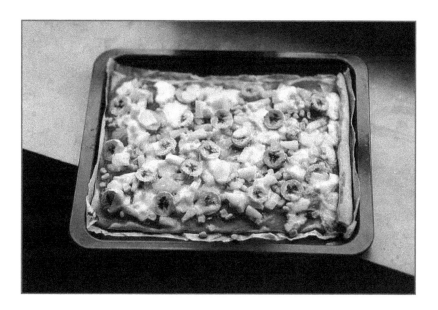

Servings:2

INGREDIENTS

- Pizza dough with tomato sauce, combination pack, filling a tray
- Tomatoes)
- ½ can Corn, approx. 280 g each
- ½ can Pineapple pieces, approx. 420 g each
- Banana (noun)
- 1 pck. Mozzarella, approx. 125 g each

PREPARATION

1.   The dough and sauce can of course also be made fresh. Recipes for this can be found in the database.

2.   Preheat the oven according to the package instructions for the pizza dough or to 200 ° C convection or 220 ° C top bottom heat. Spread the pizza dough out on a baking sheet and cover with the tomato sauce. Cut the tomato into slices and spread on the pizza. Spread the drained corn and the drained pineapple pieces on top.

3.   Also cut the banana into slices and garnish the pizza with it.

4.   Depending on how much the mozzarella is to be baked, either top the pizza directly with mozzarella and bake it or first put it in the oven without cheese for 10-15 minutes, then put the mozzarella on top and put the pizza back in the oven until it is the way you want it Tan.

Tomato canapes

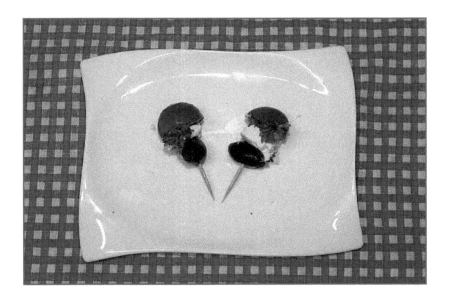

Servings:1

INGREDIENTS

- Date tomato
- 1 pinch salt and pepper
- ½ slice Goat cheese (from a roll)
- 1 pinch Herbs, Italian
- 1 sheet Basil, fresh
- Olives, green or black, pitted

PREPARATION

1   Cut the date tomato lengthways and sprinkle the cut surfaces with a little salt and pepper. Sprinkle 1/2 slice of goat cheese (thickness to taste) with the Italian herbs and place on the lower half of the tomato.

2   Place the basil leaf and the top half of the tomato on top.

3   Now fix the olive with a toothpick or cocktail stick.

4   Goes fast, tastes great and is well suited as finger food for parties.

5   The ingredients are given for 1 tomato appetizer.

Apple-ginger-lemon risotto

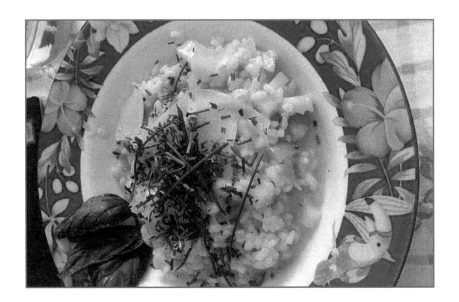

Servings:1

INGREDIENTS

- 70 g   Risotto rice
- 200 ml Vegetable broth
- 2 cm ginger
- ½ Apples
- Butter flakes
- White wine, dry, for deglazing
- ½ Lemon, zest and juice
- Hard cheese, Italian

PREPARATION

1. Rinse the lemon with hot water. Roughly chop the peel and set aside along with the lemon juice.
2. Rinse the apple and cut into coarse sticks or cubes.
3. Roast the risotto rice in the butter and deglaze with white wine and lemon juice. After deglazing, add the lemon peel. Simmer.
4. Now keep adding parts of the broth and reducing it, stirring constantly. When the rice is "soggy", turn off the stove and stir in some of the cheese.
5. The risotto is ready to serve.

Gorgonzola noodles with compote

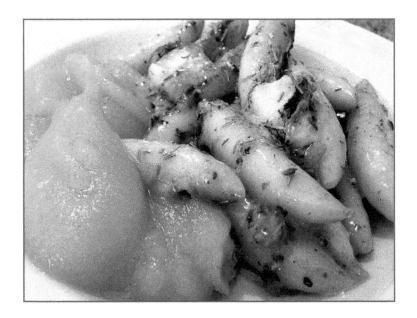

Servings: 2

INGREDIENTS

- 500 g Potato noodles
- 200 g Gorgonzola dolce
- 1 large Onion, red
- 1 glass Apple compote, ideal with a slight acidity
- pepper
- oregano
- Herbs, Italian
- 2 tbsp oil

PREPARATION

1   Heat 2 tablespoons of oil in a pan, cut the onion into small pieces and fry in it for about three minutes.

2   Add the potato noodles as well as the herbs and spices and stir.

3   Wait until the potato noodles have the desired degree of browning, then spread the Gorgonzola over it and stir well for about a minute so that it does not burn. Depending on the pan, another tablespoon of oil can also be added.

4   When the gorgonzola is not completely melted, the dish can be served. Serve with the apple compote.

5   Note: An apple compote with a slight acidity is better for my taste than a very sweet compote.

6   If you like it spiciness, you can also use some chili oil.

cheese salad

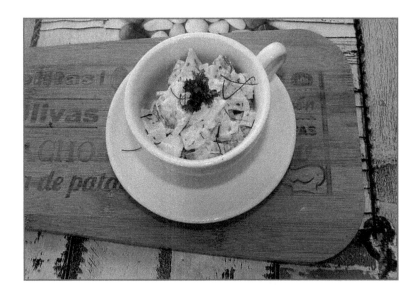

Servings:4

INGREDIENTS

- 450 g Gouda, young, in one piece
- 1 small Can Mandarin, 300 g
- ½ pck. Herbs, Italian, frozen, approx. 25 g, e.g. B. from Iglo
- 1 tbsp. Garden herbs, TK, z. B. from Iglo
- 3 tbsp, heaped Salad Cream (Miracel Whip)
- 150 ml Natural yoghurt

PREPARATION

1   Cut the cheese into small pieces.
2   Drain and chop the mandarins.
3   Mix some of the juice with the salad cream,
     natural yoghurt and herbs, then fold in the
     mandarins and cheese

Cherry chutney made from sweet cherries

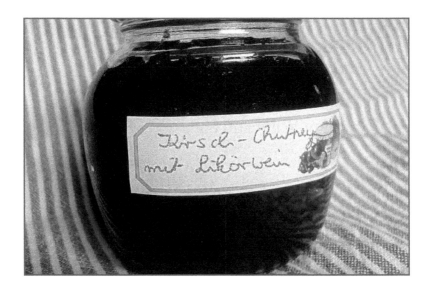

Servings:1

INGREDIENTS

- 350 g Sweet cherries, pitted, approx. 400 g gross weight
- 2 small ones Onion, red, approx. 100 g
- 2 cm Ginger, approx. 13 g, finely grated
- 100 ml Sweet wine, Italian, e.g. Marsala
- 35 ml Walnut vinegar, alternatively raspberry vinegar
- 50 g sugar
- Bay leaf

- 1 tsp, leveled Allspice powder
- 1 tsp, leveled Mustard seeds
- 1 tbsp. Coriander seeds
- ½ tsp Pul beaver
-

PREPARATION

1 Finely dice the pitted cherries and onions.
2 Mix with the remaining ingredients in a saucepan and bring to the boil on the stove. Simmer over low heat for 90 minutes.
3 The mass should boil down thickly until there is almost no liquid left.
4 Therefore stir more often, especially at the end of the cooking time.
5 Remove the bay leaf and pour the chutney into prepared sterile jars and close immediately.
6 Makes about 2 smaller glasses.

Colorful vegetable salad

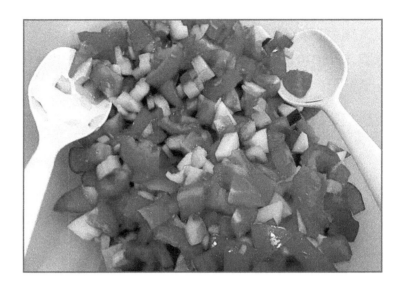

Servings:12

INGREDIENTS

For the salad:
- 8 Tomatoes
- 2 Cucumber
- 2 Bell pepper
- 2 Apples
- 4 Garlic cloves
- 400 gCheese, vegans just leave it out

For the dressing:
- 100 ml Olive oil or rapeseed oil

- 50 mlVinegar,B. Balsamic
- 1 teaspoon Honey or a suitable vegan substitute
- 1 teaspoon, heaped   mustard
- 1 teaspoon salt and pepper
- 2 Teaspoons Herbs of Provence or Italian herbs
-

PREPARATION

1   Roughly peel the cucumber and cut in half lengthways.

2   Remove the seeds with a teaspoon and then season the cucumbers with salt. After brewing for at least 15 minutes, squeeze the cucumbers out. Cucumbers contain a lot of water.

3   The pitting, salting, and squeezing will keep the lettuce from watering down.

4   Wash the tomatoes, peppers and apples and peel or core them if necessary.

5   Dice tomatoes, peppers, apples, cheese and cucumber into pieces approx. 1 cm in size. Peel and finely chop the garlic and place the ingredients in a bowl.

6   For the dressing, put the oil and vinegar in a small container.

7   You should be able to smell and taste the acid clearly.

8   So if a vinegar that is too mild is used, the ratio may have to be changed to 1: 1.

9   Whisk the oil and vinegar with the honey, mustard and spices and pour over the salad. Mix the ingredients well.

Tomato and sheep cheese salad with "whistle" as the main course

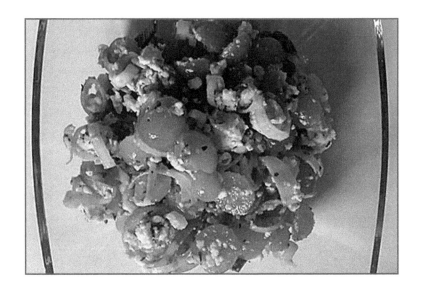

Servings:2

INGREDIENTS

- 60 Cherry tomato
- 350 g Sheep cheese or feta cheese
- ½ Vegetable onion or white sweet onion
- 150 g Blueberries, fresh
- For the dressing:
- 2 bag Seasoning mix (Knorr Salatkrönung "Italian style")
- 2 bag Seasoning mix (Knorr Salatkrönung "lamb's lettuce")

- 3 tbsp Crema di balsamic vinegar
- 2 pinch sugar
- Salt and pepper, whiter, freshly ground
- 50 mlwater
- 4 tbsp Pumpkin seed oil

Also:
- 150 g Lamb's lettuce (Rapunzel)
- 50 g Pine nuts
- Some Basil leaves

PREPARATION

1   Halve the cherry tomatoes.
2   Roughly crumble the feta with your fingers and add to the tomatoes.
3   Cut the vegetable onions into small cubes, sprinkle a little butter with a little sugar and salt to caramelize them and cook in the pan for a few minutes until the desired degree of browning.
4   Let the onion cool and mix with the tomato-feta mix, then carefully mix the blueberries with the tomato-feta mix.
5   Mix the contents of the salad coronation bags with oil, balsamic vinegar, sugar, salt, pepper and finally water (season to taste) separately.

6   Pour this sauce into the tomato and feta mix, mix everything well using a salad serving set. Tear up the lamb's lettuce a little and also mix it with the tomato and feta mix.

7   Brown the pine nuts briefly and at a high temperature in the pan without fat, turning quickly so that they don't get too dark.

8   Let the pine nuts cool and mix with the salad.

9   Top with a few shredded basil leaves.

10 This goes well with baguette z. B. with baked olives or tomatoes.

11 With 2 servings, one serving has 360 Kcal.

Hearty grape salad

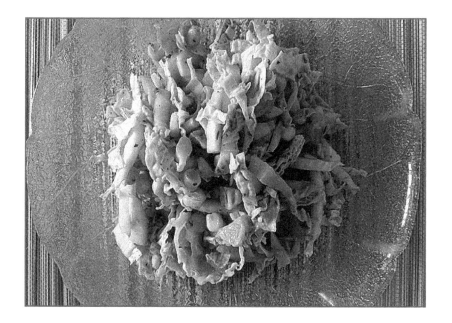

Servings:6

INGREDIENTS

- 500 g grapes
- 1 stick leek
- 1 pck. Sheep cheese
- 1 pck. Salad herbs, Italian
- 4 tbsp olive oil

PREPARATION

1	Halve the grapes.
2	Cut the leek into thin rings.
3	Crumble the cheese in your hand.
4	Add herbs and oil.
5	Mix everything together and serve.

Fresh Halloween salad

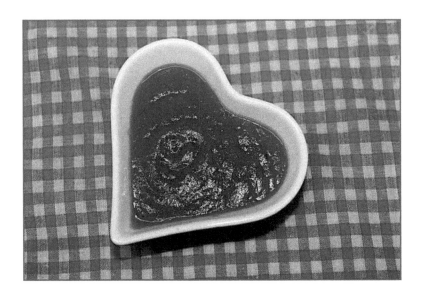

Servings:4

INGREDIENTS

- 1 head Chinese cabbage
- 1 bunch Spring onion (4 - 5 sticks)
- 1 can Corn
- 1 large Persimmons or oranges or tangerines
- 1 tbsp Balsamic vinegar
- 1 bag Herbs, Italian
- 75 ml Condensed milk
- 4 tbsp oil
- 4 tbsp water

- Something Garlic powder
-

PREPARATION

6 Wash the Chinese cabbage and drain well. Then cut into bite-sized strips. Peel and dice the persimmons.

7 Wash the spring onions well, peel them and cut them into thin slices.

8 Drain the canned corn (tip: if you want, you can use some stock for the dressing).

9 Then place in a salad bowl together with the Chinese cabbage strips, the diced persimmon and the spring onion strips.

10 For the dressing, put 75 ml of condensed milk in a measuring cup.

11 Then add 4 tablespoons of oil and 4 tablespoons of water. Mix everything together with the balsamic vinegar and the bag with Italian herbs.

12 Then season with salt, pepper and the garlic powder.

13 Pour the finished dressing evenly over the salad. Then mix everything very well and chill the salad.

14 Let it steep for about 30 minutes so that it gets the flavor it needs.

15 Tip: If you don't have persimmons at hand, you can also use diced oranges or tangerines.

Levilo's curry ketchup

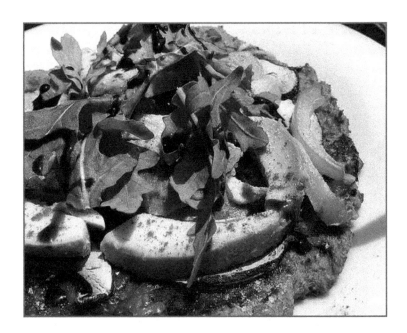

Servings:1

INGREDIENTS

- 1,000 g Tomatoes)
- 2 large Onion
- 1 large Apple
- 30 g Sugar, brown
- 1 tbsp Salt
- 1 teaspoon curry
- 100 ml Apple Cider Vinegar
- 1 tbsp Mustard medium hot
- chili

- pepper
- Herbs, Italian
- Carnation

PREPARATION

1   Chop the onions and apple and place in a saucepan with the tomatoes.
2   Add the other ingredients and cook for 20 minutes until the apple is soft.
3   Remove the clove, puree the sauce and then strain.
4   This creates the usual ketchup consistency.
5   Pour the hot sauce into clean glass containers and seal them. Turn the glasses upside down until the sauce has cooled.

Sweet potato pizza low carb

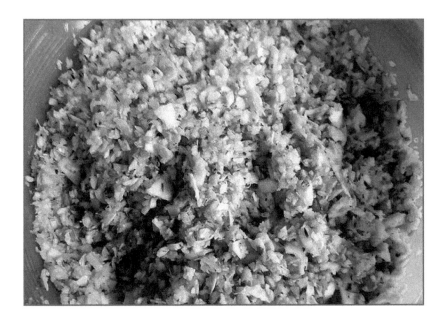

Servings:2

INGREDIENTS

- 1 large Sweet potato
- n. B.Tomato paste, flavored, or pizza tomatoes
- salt and pepper
- Herbs, Italian
- 2 tbsp Psyllium husks
- 3 tbsp Whole wheat flour
- n. B. Vegetables of your choice
- n. B. Cheese, grated
- 1 handful arugula

- Avocado

PREPARATION

1   Peel the sweet potato, cut into large cubes, cook until soft. Drain the water and puree the potato cubes. Mix in 2 tbsp phylum husks, 3 tbsp whole meal flour, salt, pepper and Italian herbs using a hand mixer.

2   Press 2 round flat cakes from the sticky dough onto baking paper and place on a baking sheet.

3   Pre-bake in a hot oven at 200 ° C top / bottom heat for 20 minutes.

4   Then add seasoned tomato paste (or pizza tomatoes) to the bottoms. Spread the cheese of your choice and vegetables (e.g. mushrooms and peppers) over the top and place in the oven for another 10 minutes. Then put the rocket and avocado in strips on top.

White cabbage salad

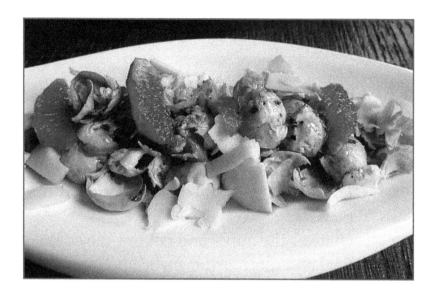

Servings:8

INGREDIENTS

- 1 kg White cabbage
- 2 m.-large Carrot
- 1 m.-large Apple
- Onion (noun)
- Garlic cloves)
- salt and pepper
- vinegar
- oil
- 4 tbsp Herbs, Italian (Tuscan spice mixture)

- 1 teaspoon mustard
- 1 teaspoon sugar
- 1 teaspoon Vegetable broth powder
- 100 ml Water, hot

PREPARATION

1   Quarter the cabbage, cut out the stalk and cut each quarter into large pieces.
2   Peel the carrots and cut them into large pieces.
3   Quarter the apple and cut out the core.
4   Peel and quarter the garlic and onion.
5   Put 1/4 of each of the ingredients in the mixing bowl and chop and transfer for 6 seconds on level 6.
6   For the sauce, add the remaining ingredients to the mixing bowl, mix and season to taste. Pour over the salad ingredients and mix.
7   Let it steep for several hours. Season again to taste.

Brussels sprouts salad with blood orange dressing

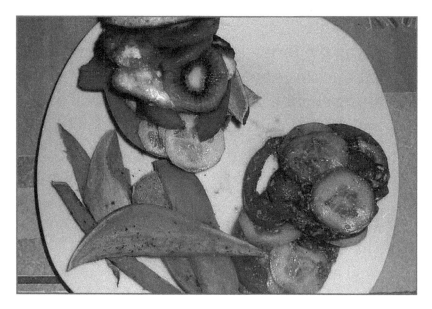

Servings: 2

INGREDIENTS

- 250 g Brussels sprouts
- Salt water
- Ice water for quenching
- 2 Blood orange
- 3 tbsp olive oil
- 3 tbsp raspberry vinegar
- 1 teaspoon honey
- 1 teaspoon Herbs, Italian, dried

- n. B. Cheese of your choice, for garnish
- Salt and pepper from the mill
-

PREPARATION

1. Clean the Brussels sprouts and carefully peel off the leaves one by one.
2. Bring about 2 liters of water to the boil in a saucepan, lightly salt and briefly blanch the leaves in it.
3. If possible, chill in ice water, then drain well in a sieve.
4. Otherwise, pour the leaves into a sieve and rinse carefully with cold water.
5. Peel a blood orange.
6. The white skin must be completely gone. Then fillet.
7. Squeeze out the second blood orange and put 5 tablespoons of juice for the dressing in a bowl. Add olive oil, raspberry vinegar, honey and herbs to the juice and stir well. Season to taste with salt and pepper.
8. Divide the Brussels sprouts on two plates. Cut the cheese into slightly wider strips and placc the orange fillets on top. Spread the dressing over it.

Kiwi halloumi burger

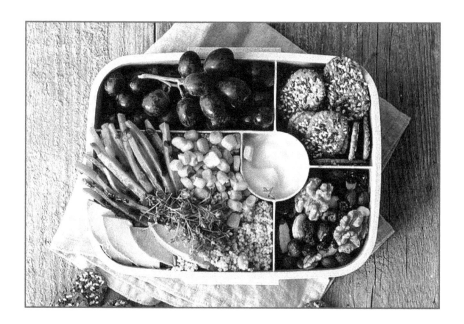

Servings:4

INGREDIENTS
- 4 Burgerbun
- 250 g Halloumi
- 2 Sweet potato
- 4 Tomatoes
- Cucumber
- Kiwi
- 20 g Hard cheese, Italian
- 40 ml mayonnaise
- 10 ml Pumpkin seed oil
- 1 tbsp vinegar

- Something salt and pepper
- 1 tbsp Butter for toasting the rolls
- 2 tbsp Oil for frying the halloumi

PREPARATION

1 Set the oven to 220 degrees top-bottom heat. Peel the kiwi and cucumber.
2 Cut the halloumi into 1 cm thick slices.
3 Halve the tomatoes and remove the stalk. Then cut the kiwi and tomatoes into 0.5 cm thick slices and the cucumber into 1 cm cubes. Peel the sweet potato and cut into 0.5 cm thick wedges, pat them dry with kitchen paper.
4 Place the sweet potatoes on a baking sheet lined with baking paper, sprinkle neatly with salt and pepper and bake on the middle rack in the oven for 15-20 minutes.
5 Cut the buns. Heat the butter in a pan on medium heat.
6 Brown the rolls with the cut surface facing down for 2 - 3 minutes, take them out and set them aside for a moment.
7 Heat the oil in the same pan and fry the halloumi until golden brown.
8 Grate the hard cheese. In a large bowl, mix the pumpkin seed oil, vinegar, salt and pepper to make a dressing.

9 Mix half of the tomato slices, the cucumber cubes and the grated hard cheese into the dressing.

10 Spread some mayonnaise on the bun halves. Top the rolls with the sliced halloumi, the kiwi, the remaining tomatoes and a few wedges of sweet potatoes.

11 Serve the finished burger with the lettuce and the remaining sweet potato wedges.

12 The burger and its side dishes contain approx. 796 Kcal per serving.

Buddha Bowl lunch box with break crackers

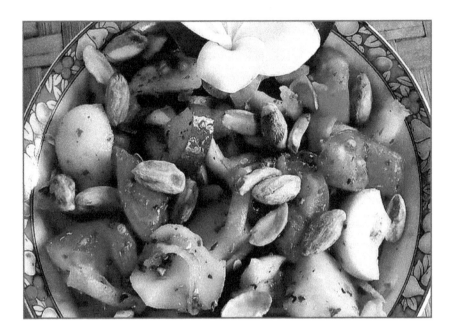

Servings:1

INGREDIENTS
- 10 Saltlett's Break Cracker
- 1 small Carrot
- 1 small Onion (noun)
- 2 Teaspoons Rapeseed oil
- 100 g millet
- 200 ml Vegetable broth
- salt and pepper
- Chilli powder
- ginger

- Curry powder
- Herbs, Italian
- Something Lemon juice, fresher
- ½ Avocado
- 5 tbsp Coconut yogurt (yogurt alternative)
- Something orange juice
- 4 tbsp Corn
- Cress, fresh, at will
- n. B. grapes
- n. B. Ready mix (nut and grape mix)

PREPARATION

1. Peel the carrot, cut in half and cut into thin strips.
Peel the onion and cut into small pieces.
Fry both in a little rapeseed oil for a few minutes.
Place on a plate and set aside.
2. Put the millet in the same pan and add 200 ml of vegetable stock.
Bring to the boil and simmer for about seven minutes, until the millet is soft and has absorbed the liquid. Season well.
3. Cut the avocado into large pieces.
4. Season the coconut yoghurt with a little orange juice, salt and pepper.
5. Now arrange everything in the lunch box. Spread the crackers, grapes, nut and grape mixture and yoghurt on the compartments.

Put the millet in the largest compartment and distribute the avocado, corn and carrot.
Finally sprinkle the fresh cress over the Buddha Bowl.

Mixed salad with honeydew melon and avocado

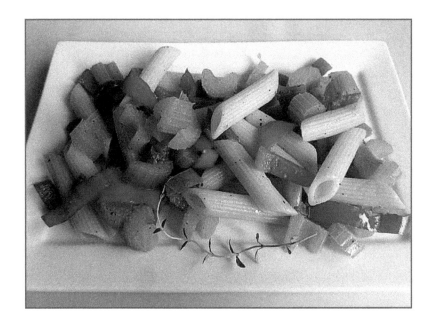

Servings:2

INGREDIENTS

- 4 m.-large Tomato, fully ripe
- 1 small Cucumber, slim
- 6 small Onion, red
- ½ Avocado, ripe
- ½ Honeydew melon, fully ripe
- ¼ Carrot

For the dressing:
- 2 Teaspoons Salt or chicken broth, instant

- 1 tbsp, heaped Herbs, Italian
- ½ tsp Macis powder, alternatively freshly grated nutmeg
- 1 teaspoon Pepper, black, freshly ground
- 1 pinch Chilli Powder (Chipotle)
- 1 teaspoon Sugar, white
- 2 m.-large Garlic clove (s), fresh
- 2 tbsp Red wine vinegar
- 2 tbsp orange juice
- 6 tbsp Extra virgin olive oil
- To garnish:
- n. B. Pistachio nuts
- n. B. Flowers and leaves
-

PREPARATION

1   Wash fruits and vegetables and chop them up to size. Peel and roughly grate the carrot, peel the onions and cut across into 2 mm thick slices. Quarter the cucumber lengthways and cut across into 5 mm thick slices. Halve the avocado, remove the core and use a ball cutter to cut out hemispheres from one half. Cut 3 approx. 1 cm thick slices crosswise from a pitted half of the honeydew melon, peel and cut into approx. 1 x 1 cm cubes. Squeeze the tomatoes.

2   Sprinkle the ingredients from instant chicken broth to sugar for dressing over the salad, mix and let ripen for 10 minutes. Peel and squeeze the garlic cloves and mix with the vinegar and orange juice.

3   Add the vinegar mixture and the olive oil to the salad just before serving. Spread the salad on the serving plates, garnish and serve with white bread.

Vegetarian macaroni with fig and pepper sauce

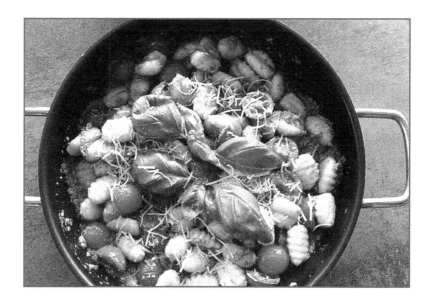

Servings:4

INGREDIENTS

- 400 gmacaroni
- For the sauce:
- 4 tbsp olive oil
- Salt and pepper from the mill
- 6th Bell pepper, red and green
- 1 stick Celery
- 3 Fig, ripe

PREPARATION

1   For the sauce, cut the peppers in half and remove the stems and seeds. Also remove the white partitions, then wash the pods and drain well.

2   Clean, wash and drain the celery. Cut both ingredients into fine cubes or strips.

3   Heat the olive oil in a pan, add the vegetables and cook for about 10 minutes. Stir every now and then, adding a little water if necessary. Season to taste with salt and pepper.

4   Peel the figs, cut into small pieces and stir into the vegetable sauce.

5   Keep the sauce warm.

6   Cook the macaroni in plenty of salted water according to the instructions on the packet, then pour them onto a sieve and drain.

7   Mix the macaroni with the fig sauce before serving.

Gnocchi with avocado and basil pesto

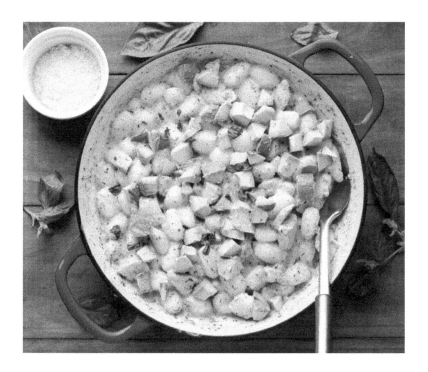

Servings:6

INGREDIENTS

- 1,200 g Gnocchi, homemade or from the cooling shelf
- 2 federal government Basil, roughly chopped
- 2 Avocado
- 8 tbsp olive oil
- 350 g Cherry tomato
- 100 g Ground almonds

- Lemon, juice of it
- 2 toe garlic
- 100 g Parmesan
- 2 pinch sugar
- salt and pepper
- Butter for frying
-

PREPARATION

1. Halve the avocados, remove the stone and remove the pulp from the skin.
2. Peel the garlic cloves and finely puree them with the avocado pulp, basil, lemon juice, almonds and olive oil. Season to taste with salt and pepper.
3. Heat the butter in a pan and fry the gnocchi until golden brown. Set aside and keep warm.
4. Halve the cherry tomatoes, heat a little butter in a pan and add the tomato halves with the sugar.
5. Reduce the heat, then add the avocado pesto and gnocchi and mix well. Season to taste with salt and pepper.
6. Grate the parmesan.
7. Arrange the gnocchi on plates and serve sprinkled with parmesan.

Risotto with green asparagus and parmesan

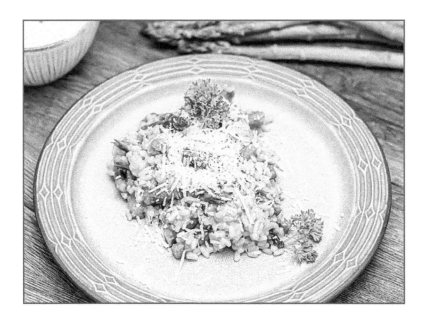

Servings:4

INGREDIENTS

- 500 gAsparagus, green
- Salt and pepper, freshly ground
- 1 pinch sugar
- 2 Shallot
- 3 tbsp butter
- 300 gRisotto rice
- 100 ml White wine, dry or water
- 800 ml Veal stock, hotter
- 3 stems Parsley smooth
- 75 g   Parmesan

PREPARATION

1   Rinse the asparagus and break off the bottom. Peel the asparagus spears on the lower third and cut into 3 cm long pieces. Bring about half a liter of salted water with sugar to the boil and cook the asparagus pieces in it for eight to ten minutes over a low heat. Drain on a sieve.

2   Peel and dice the shallots.

3   Heat half of the butter and sauté the shallots over medium heat until translucent.

4   Add the rice and cook until translucent while stirring (do not brown!).

5   Pour in the wine and stir until it has evaporated. Add a good shot of hot veal stock to the rice and cook in an open saucepan over a low heat for about 20 minutes. Stir occasionally and keep adding a little stock so that the rice is always just covered with liquid. At the end the risotto should have a creamy consistency.

6   Carefully stir in asparagus pieces, remaining butter, 40 g grated Parmesan and chopped parsley. Season the risotto with salt and pepper. Scatter the rest of the grated parmesan on top and serve the risotto immediately.

Coconut - panna cotta

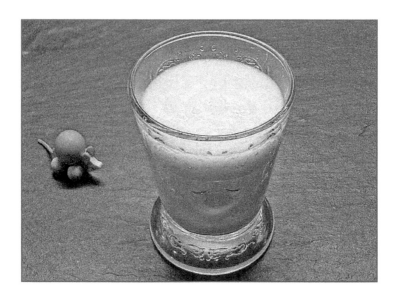

Servings:4
INGREDIENTS
- 2 tbsp sugar
- 250 ml Coconut milk
- 250 ml cream
- 3 sheets gelatin
- Fruit of your choice
-

PREPARATION

1   Soak the gelatine in cold water. Stir in
    coconut milk, cream and sugar, bring to the
    boil and simmer gently for a few minutes.

Squeeze out the gelatine and dissolve it in the hot cream mixture.

2   Let it set in the refrigerator (approx. 3-4 hours) and serve upside down or as a dumpling with fresh fruit.

3   If you like it more "snappy", you can stir some roasted coconut flakes into the mixture.

4   Then after about 1 hour of cooling time you should stir again so that the coconut flakes are evenly distributed.

Lemon polenta

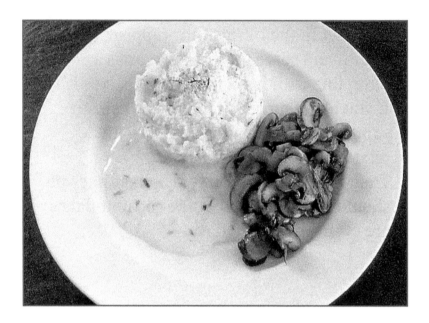

Servings:4

INGREDIENTS

- 200 gpolenta
- 300 ml milk
- 500 ml vegetable stock
- 50 g butter
- Lemon, untreated, the juice of half the fruit and the whole zest)
- 1 tbsp Thyme, torn leaves
- ½ tsp coriander
- salt and pepper

PREPARATION

1   Bring the milk with the vegetable stock to the boil, pour in the polenta, stir well and bring to the boil.

2   Take the pot off the stove and let the polenta soak for about 30 minutes (or according to the instructions on the package).

3   Stir in butter, thyme, coriander, lemon juice and the finely chopped zest and season with salt and pepper.

4   Tastes good with pan-fried food.

Fennel salad with oranges

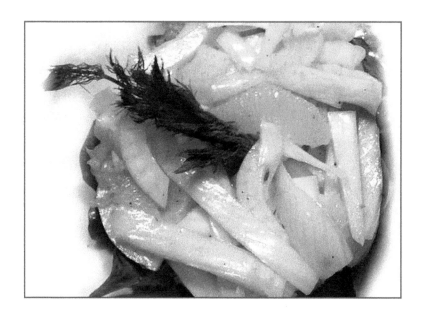

Servings:1

INGREDIENTS
- ½ Fennel bulb
- Orange
- 1 handful Lettuce, green, rocket or lamb's lettuce
- 1 tbsp olive oil
- 2 tbsp White wine vinegar, fruity
- ¼ tsp Mustard, hotter
- salt and pepper

PREPARATION

1 Halve the fennel without the green and stem and remove the stalk and outer leaves if they no longer look crisp.
2 Then rinse the halves under running water and dry a little. Cut the fennel into as thin slices as possible.
3 Fillet the orange and collect the juice.
4 Mix the orange juice with the olive oil, white wine vinegar, a little hot mustard, salt and pepper well with a fork or whisk.
5 Add the orange fillets and the fennel, let it steep a little and arrange on a bed of lettuce.

Fruity mascarpone cream

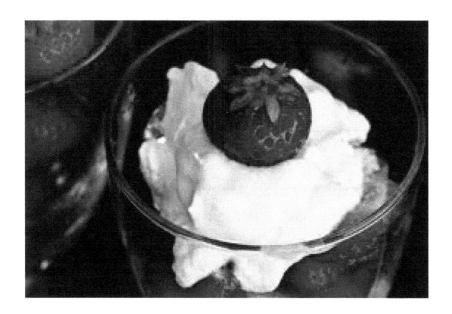

Servings:6

INGREDIENTS

- 750 g Raspberries
- 10 tbsp Orange liqueur
- 500 gMascarpone
- 500 glow fat quark
- 150 g powdered sugar
- 8 tbsp Lemon juice
- 100 ml Coffee, boiled, cold
- 2 bottle Butter-vanilla flavor
- n. B. Grated chocolate

PREPARATION

1   Mix the mascarpone, quark, powdered
     sugar, lemon juice, coffee and vanilla flavor
     until smooth.
2   Put half of the fruit in a bowl and pour half
     of the mascarpone cream over it.
3   Repeat the whole thing. Smooth the cream
     and sprinkle chocolate flakes over the cream
     as required.

Il Caviale di Belzebù al Limone

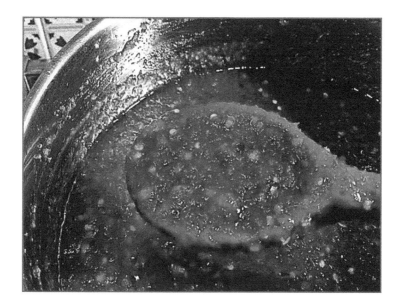

Servings:1

INGREDIENTS

- 5 kg Lemon, fully ripe, untreated and unsprayed)
- 1 kg Honey, (linden)
- 180 g Chilli pepper, Calabrian
-

PREPARATION

4   Peel the lemons, cut the peel into thin strips, and then work these into cubes with an edge length of around 2 mm. Now peel the lemons

a second time and roughly chop them. We need the white to gel.

5   Halve the lemons and squeeze out the juice.
6   In a saucepan, cook the white peels and juice until the peels are soft.
7   Then puree finely. Now add the raw cubes to the puree and also add the honey and chillies. Bring everything to the boil, stirring constantly, until the desired consistency is achieved. Due to the consistency, it is advisable to wear long, thick gloves and protective goggles.
8   Then pour into jars that have been boiled hot and close.

Rocket with orange fillets

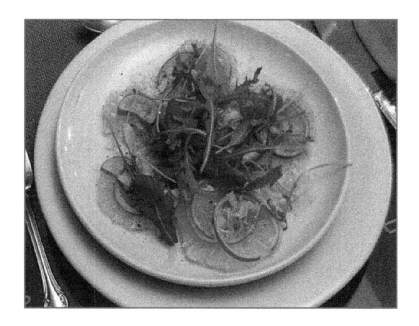

Servings:4

INGREDIENTS
- 2 large Orange
- 1 large Onion (s), red
- 1 bunch Arugula, without stems
- 150 g Parmesan
- 8 tbsp olive oil
- Balsamic cream
- Salt and pepper, from the mill

PREPARATION

- Wash the rocket and remove it from the stems. Peel the oranges so that the white skin is completely removed.
- Then cut into thin slices.
- Cut the red onion into thin rings. Slice the parmesan.
- Place the orange slices in a circle on the plate, place onion rings on top.
- Sprinkle the rocket on top and spread the parmesan on top.
- Season with salt and pepper, drizzle with olive oil and garnish generously with balsamic cream.

Panna cotta with strawberry sauce

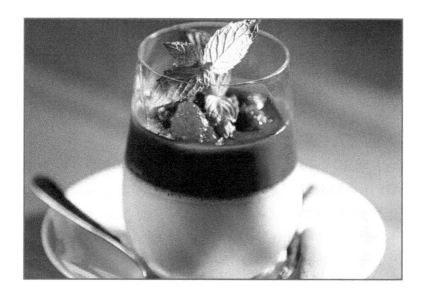

Servings:4

INGREDIENTS

- 400 gcream
- Vanilla pod
- 50 g sugar
- 3 sheets Gelatin, white
- For the sauce:
- 400 g Strawberries
- 50 g sugar

PREPARATION

- Bring the cream with the sugar and the sliced vanilla pod to the boil and simmer for about 15 minutes while stirring.
- Soak the gelatine in cold water.
- Remove the vanilla pod from the cream and dissolve the squeezed gelatin in the cream.
- Rinse the molds with cold water, pour in the cream and leave to set in the refrigerator for at least 2 hours.
- Wash and clean the strawberries and puree them with the sugar.
- Brush through a sieve.
- Remove the panna cotta from the molds and serve with the strawberry sauce.

Orange salad

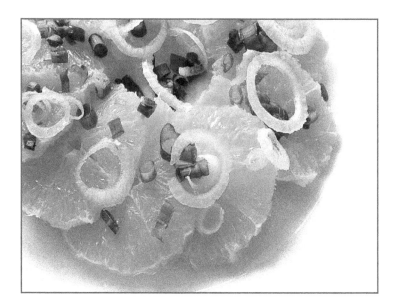

Servings:4

INGREDIENTS

- 4 Orange
- 1 small Onion, red
- 2 Spring onion
- 6 tbsp olive oil
- 2 tbsp Balsamic or lemon juice
- 5 tbsp orange juice
- Something pepper

PREPARATION

- Peel the oranges and cut them into slices.
- Also cut the onion into slices.
- Place oranges and onions decoratively on a deep plate.
- Scatter pepper over the top and drizzle with oil, vinegar and orange juice.
- Cut the spring onions into rings and sprinkle over them.
- Cover with foil and leave in the refrigerator for 2 hours.

Amarena cherry jam

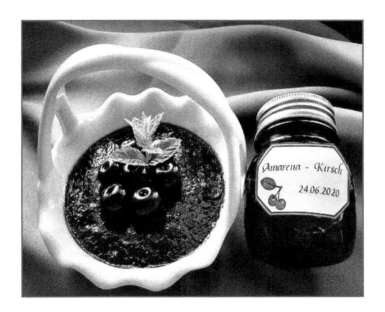

Servings:1

INGREDIENTS

- 400 gCherry, pitted (e.g. heart cherries)
- 100 ml Amaretto
- 250 g Preserving sugar
- 1 pck.vanilla sugar
- 1 splash Bitter almond flavor
- 1 splash Flavor (vanilla flavor)

PREPARATION

1   Put all ingredients in a high saucepan, bring to the boil and simmer for about 15 minutes over medium heat, then puree.

2   Put a full teaspoon on a cold plate for the gelling test.

3   If the jam is firm, it can now be poured into cold rinsed glasses. Screw on glasses immediately.

4   If you don't like the jam too firm, you can add a little more amaretto if you like.

Rocket salad with caramelized pears, blue cheese and pine nuts

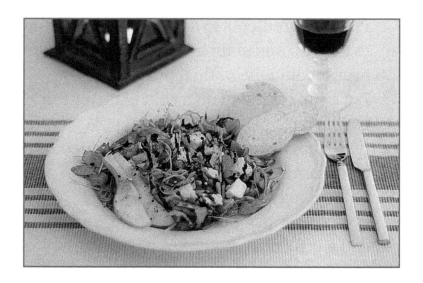

Servings:4

INGREDIENTS

- 160 g arugula
- 3 Pear
- 300 gBlue cheese
- 100 g Pine nuts
- 30 g butter
- 2 tbsp sugar
- 1 shotBalsamic vinegar
- 1 pinch salt

- 1 pinch pepper

PREPARATION

1 This salad fits perfectly into a 3-course menu, but can also be eaten for dinner with two slices of baguette and a glass of red wine.
2 Wash the rocket and drain well.
3 Quarter the pears and cut into slices.
4 Incidentally, roast the pine nuts in a pan until they are nice and brown.
5 Melt the butter in a pan, then add the sugar and caramelize.
6 Deglaze everything with balsamic vinegar and fry the pears for about 2-3 minutes on both sides.
7 Finally, cut the blue cheese into cubes and arrange on the bed of rocket with the pears and pine nuts.
8 Season to taste with salt and pepper.
9 It goes well with baguette and red wine.

Triangles of cheese

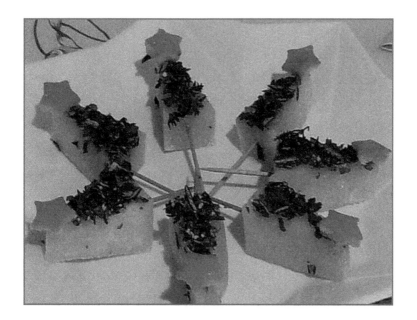

Servings:6

INGREDIENTS

- Pecorino in one piece
- 300 ghoney
- 30 g Herbs, fresh, e.g. B. parsley, rosemary, thyme
- Pepper, green
- Berries, pink
- Orange

PREPARATION

- Cut the cheese into triangles and remove the crust.
- Put the spices in a bowl and coarsely chop them together with the green pepper and pink berries.
- Wash and peel the orange, remove the whites and use a cookie cutter to cut out small stars.
- Brush one side of the cheese, brush with honey and sprinkle with herbs and pepper.
- Put a skewer on the lower half, e.g. B. glue a toothpick and the orange star to the top with a little honey so that it sticks.
- In this way, the cheese nibbles form little trees.

Field salad with oranges

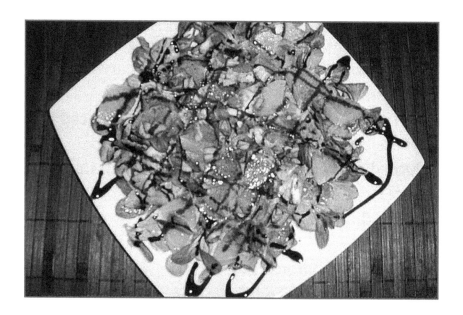

Servings:2

INGREDIENTS

- 1 bowl Lamb's lettuce
- 2 Orange
- ½ Onion
- salt and pepper
- Balsamic vinegar
- olive oil
- Balsamico - Glassa

PREPARATION

- Wash the lamb's lettuce thoroughly, remove the small roots, drain the water and then arrange the lamb's lettuce on a plate.
- Peel and quarter the oranges, slice the quarters across a bowl and add to the lamb's lettuce. Spread the resulting juice on the salad in the bowl.
- Finely dice half the onion and sprinkle over the salad.
- Season with salt and pepper.
- Season to taste with balsamic vinegar and olive oil.
- Decorate with balsamic glassa or another crema di balsamic vinegar.

Neapolitan orange salad

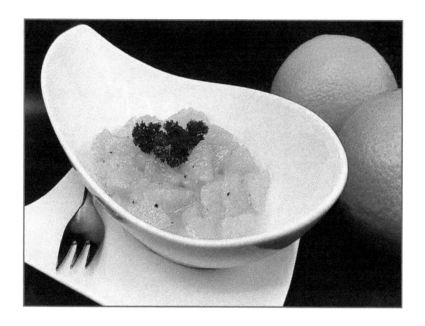

Servings:2

INGREDIENTS

- 4 large Orange, juicy sweetness
- 2 tbsp Olive oil, good quality
- Sea salt from the mill
- pepper from the grinder

PREPARATION

1   Peel the oranges and cut into bite-sized
    pieces.

2   Mix the orange pieces with the olive oil in a bowl, season with salt and pepper and season to taste.
3   Let the salad stand for 10 minutes before serving.

Pear Tiramisu

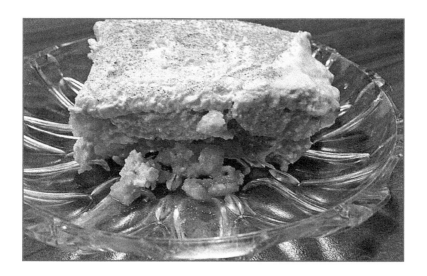

Servings:1

INGREDIENTS

- 200 gLadyfingers
- 100 ml Pear juice, 100%
- 500 gMascarpone
- 200 gWhipped cream
- 150 g Natural yoghurt, mild, 3.5% fat content
- 4th Pear, ripe, z. B. Williams Christ
- 4 tbsp sugar
- 4 tbsp cinnamon

PREPARATION

1 Place the sponge fingers in a baking dish with the sugared side down and drizzle 1 tbsp of the pear juice over each one.

2 Mix the mascarpone with 2 - 3 tablespoons of pear juice and the yogurt. Whip the whipped cream until stiff and fold it carefully into the mascarpone mixture.

3 Now distribute half of the cream evenly on the ladyfingers.

4 Wash the pears, cut in half, peel, core and cut into thin wedges.

5 Spread the pear wedges on the cream until a closed pear top is formed. Now put another layer of ladyfingers on top and drizzle with 1 tablespoon of the pear juice each time. Spread the rest of the cream evenly on the biscuits.

6 Mix the sugar with the cinnamon and use a small sieve to spread over the cream.

7 Put the finished tiramisu in a cool place and leave it to stand overnight.

Panna cotta

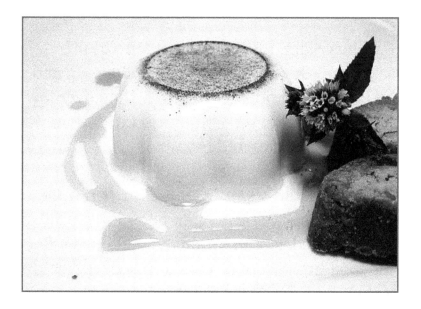

Servings:8

INGREDIENTS

- 400 gcream
- 600 ml milk
- 100 g sugar
- 2 Vanilla pod
- 8 sheets Gelatin, white
- 400 gCurrants, raspberries and blackberries
- 4 tbsp sugar

PREPARATION

1. Put the cream, milk and sugar (100 g) in a saucepan. Stir in the scraped vanilla pulp and add the empty pods. Bring to the boil over low heat and simmer for 15 minutes (attention: if the mixture simmered too weakly, the panna cotta will not set!) Soak the
2. gelatine in cold water. Remove the pan from the heat, remove the vanilla pods and stir in the squeezed gelatin until it has dissolved. Pour the food into 8 soufflé molds rinsed with cold water and leave to set overnight in the refrigerator.
3. Wash the berries, remove any bad spots and stalk, cut into small pieces and heat with 4 tablespoons of sugar and let simmer.
4. Tip the panna cotta out of the molds (cut all around with a warm knife or hold the mold briefly in hot water if it doesn't work). Garnish with the berry compote.

Tagliatelle with tomato and pepper sauce

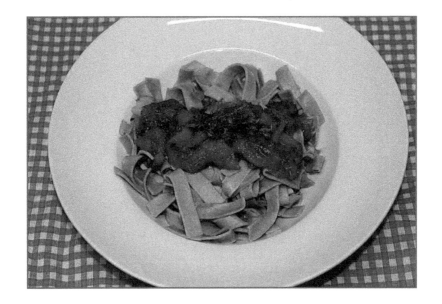

Servings:4

INGREDIENTS

- 2 Bell pepper
- Chilli pepper
- Onion (noun)
- 1 can Tomato, organic, chopped
- 500 gTagliatelle
- 2 tbsp olive oil
- 1 tbsp Tomato paste
- 150 ml orange juice

- salt
- pepper

PREPARATION

1   Wash, halve and core the peppers.
2   Bake in the preheated oven at 250 ° C under the grill until the shell throws black bases. This takes about 10-12 minutes. Take out of the oven and cover with a damp cloth. The skin can then be easily peeled off. Cut the peppers into cubes.
3   Cook the noodles in plenty of salted water until they are firm to the bite (1 liter of water + 1 tablespoon of salt per 100 g of noodles, approx. 7 minutes).
4   Finely dice the onion and chilli pepper and sauté in hot oil.
5   Add the tomato paste and deglaze with orange juice. Add the canned tomatoes and diced paprika. Season with salt and pepper.
6   Drain the pasta and serve with the sauce. Sprinkle with freshly grated Parmesan if you like and add a few leaves of basil.

Schwarzplentene Riebler

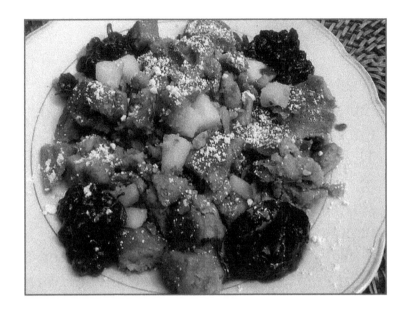

Servings:3

INGREDIENTS

- 200 g Buckwheat flour
- 250 ml milk
- 3 Egg
- 2 Apples
- ½ tsp, worked salt
- 50 g butter
- n. B. Powdered sugar (powdered sugar)
- 1 glass Cranberries

PREPARATION

1. Mix the buckwheat flour with the milk and let it soak for 1 hour.
2. Stir in the eggs one by one and add salt.
3. Melt 30 g butter in the pan.
4. Bake the rubbing mass in it, then turn and cut into pieces.
5. Continue frying and dividing until you have small pieces.
6. Peel the apples, cut into cubes, add with the remaining butter and continue frying.
7. Sprinkle the raspberry with icing sugar and serve with wild cranberries.

Refreshing summer salad with watermelon and rocket

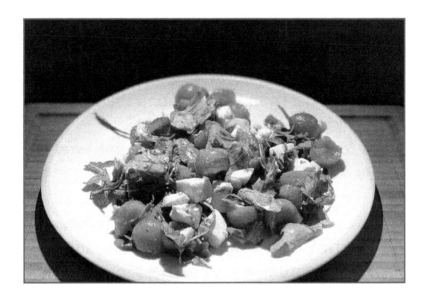

Servings:2

INGREDIENTS

- 2 tbsp Pumpkin seeds
- 400 gMelon (n), (watermelon)
- 125 g Mozzarella
- 80 g arugula
- Something salt
- Something Pepper from the grinder
- 1 teaspoon honey
- 2 tbsp Balsamic vinegar, whiter

- 2 tbsp oil

PREPARATION

1   Roast the pumpkin seeds in a pan without fat and allow to cool.

2   Cut the watermelon into cubes or use a melon cutter to cut out balls.

3   Dice the mozzarella.

4   Clean, wash and dry the rocket on kitchen paper and, if necessary, pluck it into small pieces.

5   Prepare a marinade with the remaining ingredients, season to taste and mix everything together.

Strawberry tiramisu

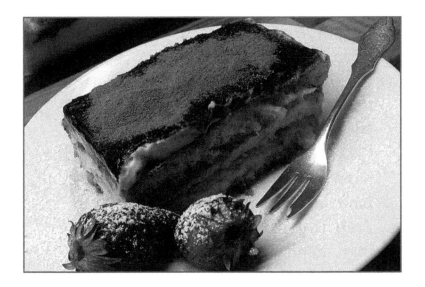

Servings:6

INGREDIENTS

- 2 pck. Custard powder
- ½ liter milk
- 60 g Sugar, (also works less)
- 1 kg   Strawberries or any berries (to taste)
- Sugar, to taste
- Something Lemon juice
- 1 cup cream
- 500 g Quark (low-fat quark)
- 125 g Sugar, rather a little less

- 400 gLadyfingers
- Cocoa powder, to sieve
-

PREPARATION

1   Mix the custard powder in a little cold milk,
    bring the rest of the milk to the boil with the
    sugar.
2   Pour the mixed pudding powder into the
    boiling milk and bring to the boil while
    stirring.
3   Let the pudding cool down, stirring
    occasionally.
4   Wash (thaw) the berries / strawberries,
    drain very well and remove the stalk (if the
    E. is fresh). Cut the fruit into small pieces
    and add sugar to taste.
5   Cover with a little lemon juice and cover with
    the juice. Then puree.
6   Whip the cream until stiff, stir the quark
    with the sugar until creamy. Gradually stir in
    the cooled pudding.
7   Fold in the stiff cream.
8   Dip the ladyfingers briefly in the strawberry
    puree and lay them out in a large casserole
    dish (25x40 cm), cover with a layer of vanilla
    cream and dip the next ladyfingers in the
    strawberry / berry puree and place over

them. Spread the rest of the cream over everything and smooth the surface. Sprinkle the cocoa on top.

9   Let it steep in the fridge for at least an hour or prepare for the next day and then put it in the fridge.

Burrata and tomatoes on avocado mirror

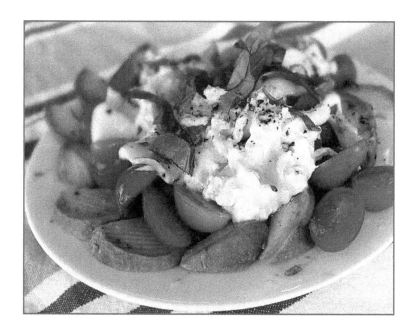

Servings:2

INGREDIENTS

- Avocado
- 220 g Tomato, yellow and red
- 100 g Burrata
- 1 teaspoon Pine nuts
- n. B. Sea salt, coarse
- n. B. pepper from the grinder
- 3 tbsp Olive oil, good
- Something Honey, more liquid
- 1 tbsp Lemon juice

- 6 Basil leaves

PREPARATION

1. Quarter the avocado, carefully remove and core the skin, cut into thin slices and fan out on a flat plate.
2. Also cut the tomatoes into slices, remove the stalk if necessary and drape on the avocado.
3. Roughly cut the burrata and place in the center of the plate.
4. Drizzle with the olive oil and lemon juice and drip some honey on top, but be careful not to take too much, salt and pepper.
5. Roast the pine nuts in a pan without fat until they are fragrant and browned.
6. Meanwhile, cut the basil into small pieces and distribute it on the plate along with the pine nuts.
7. Fresh white bread goes well with it.

Peaches filled with amaretti

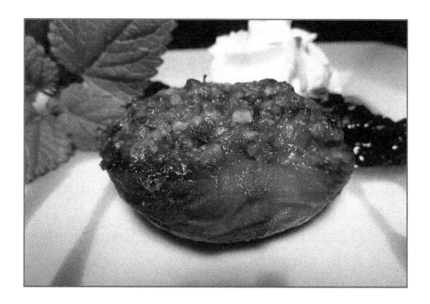

Servings:4

INGREDIENTS

- 4 Peach, ripe
- 60 g Biscuit, amoretti (pastry)
- 50 g sugar
- 40 g Almond, peeled
- 30 g butter
- 70 g Wine, muscat wine, sherry or port wine
- egg yolk
- 1 teaspoon Cocoa powder

PREPARATION

1   Cut the peaches in half and remove the stone.

2   Using a teaspoon, carefully remove some of the pulp to make a nice round opening and set it aside.

3   Drizzle the peach halves with a little lemon juice.

4   Finely crumble the amaretti and finely chop the almonds.

5   In a bowl, mix the almonds, amaretti, 20g sugar, cocoa, egg yolks and peach meat well.

6   Pour the mixture into the peach halves.

7   Preheat the oven to 200 °.

8   Brush a baking dish with butter and put the peach halves in with the filling facing up. Sprinkle with the remaining sugar and drizzle the wine, port or sherry over it.

9   Put in the oven and cook for 35 minutes. From time to time sprinkle with the escaping liquid.

10   You can serve them directly in the baking dish.

Lemon salad

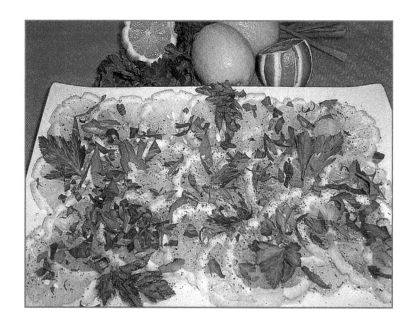

Servings:2

INGREDIENTS

- 3 Lemon, untreated organic, unpeeled
- n. B. Parsley, smooth
- salt
- Pepper from the grinder
- Extra virgin oil

PREPARATION

1   Wash the lemons with warm water.
2   Notch lengthways with a fluting knife, then cut into thin slices.
3   Arrange the lemons on a plate.
4   Season with salt and pepper from the mill, drizzle with oil.
5   Sprinkle with the coarsely chopped parsley.

Lukewarm salad of May turnips, pear and mini romaine

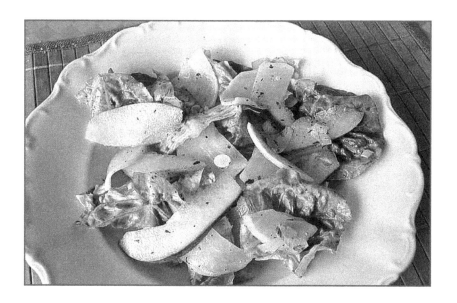

Servings:4

INGREDIENTS

For the salad:
- 2 May turnips
- Pear, (not too soft)
- Spring onion, thinly sliced
- Romaine lettuce, mini
- ½ fret Parsley, smooth, finely chopped with stems
- 1 tbsp butter

- 3 tbsp Vegetable stock, or vegetable broth
- n. B.salt and pepper
- For the vinaigrette:
- 3 tbsp White wine vinegar, or white balsamic vinegar
- 4 tbsp Olive oil, extra virgin cold-pressed
- ½ tsp Mustard, medium hot
- 1 tbsp honey
- 2 tbsp Vegetable stock, or vegetable broth
- n. B.Chilli flakes, 1 to 3 knife points

PREPARATION

6   First, the ingredients for the salad are prepared:

7   the turnips are peeled, halved and cut into slices. The pear is peeled, quartered, the core removed and also cut into slices.

8   The parsley is washed and roughly cut.

9   Wash the spring onions and cut into thin slices. The mini-romana is cut down from the tip at 5 mm intervals (down to the stalk).

10   Now the butter is heated in a non-stick pan (medium heat). The turnips, pears, spring onions and parsley are then sautéed in the heated butter for about 3 minutes, swirling frequently. Now add the stock and simmer until the stock has completely evaporated.

Swing through once or twice. Now season with salt / pepper, set aside and let cool down.

11   Preparation of the vinaigrette:

12   Put all ingredients in a mixing vessel and mix thoroughly with the hand blender. Let it infuse briefly and then mix vigorously again.

13   "Marriage" of salad and vinaigrette:

14   Put the slightly more than lukewarm contents of the pan in a salad bowl and add the sliced romaine.

15   Pour the vinaigrette over it, mix everything well with the salad servers and leave to marinate for 5 minutes. Now season again with salt and pepper according to your personal taste. Finished.

16   If you don't like a 'lukewarm' salad, just let the pan and its contents cool down completely.

Crispy bruschetta with goat cheese and strawberrie

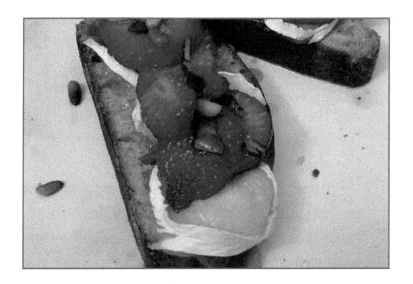

Servings:4

INGREDIENTS

- 8 slice ciabatta
- 175 g Goat cheese (brie)
- 200 gStrawberries, fresh
- 8 sheets basil
- 1 tbsp Balsamic vinegar, good one
- 1 tbsp honey
- 30 g Cashew nuts or pine nuts

PREPARATION

1 Wash and clean the strawberries and cut into thin slices.
2 Roughly chop the nuts and briefly toast them in a coated pan. Rinse the basil while wet and cut finely.
3 Carefully mix the strawberries with honey, balsamic vinegar, basil and nuts and leave to steep for 15 minutes.
4 Preheat oven to 175 degrees.
5 Roast the ciabatta slices briefly in the oven for about 5 minutes, then cover with the sliced goat cheese and bake for another 10 minutes.
6 Take the ciabatta goat cheese slices out of the oven and cover with the prepared strawberries.

Fennel and orange salad

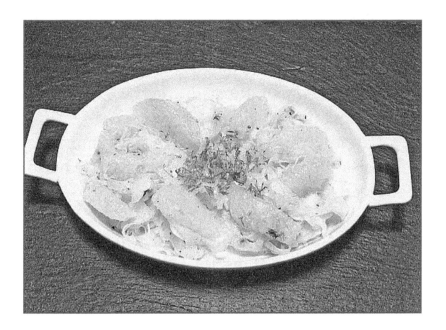

Servings:4

INGREDIENTS

- 1 bulb fennel
- Orange
- Onion, red
- 3 tbsp Fennel - green
- 3 tbsp olive oil
- salt and pepper

PREPARATION

1. Wash the fennel and cut into thin slices.
2. Peel the orange, remove the white skins and cut into thin slices.
3. Cut the onion into rings. Finely chop the fennel leaves.
4. Put all ingredients in a bowl and mix with olive oil.
5. Season with salt and pepper.
6. So that the salad can develop its full taste, it should be left covered for half a day before consumption and stirred every now and then.

CONCLUSIONS

A vegetarian diet focuses on eating vegetables. This includes dried fruits, vegetables, peas and beans, grains, seeds, and nuts. There is no single type of vegetarian diet.

Vegetarian diets continue to grow in popularity. The reasons for following a vegetarian diet are varied and include health benefits, such as reduced risk of heart disease, diabetes, and some types of cancer. However, some vegetarians consume too many processed foods, which can be high in calories, sugar, fat, and sodium, and may not consume enough fruits, vegetables, whole grains, and foods rich in calcium, missing out on the nutrients they provide.

However, with a little planning, a vegetarian diet can meet the needs of people of all ages, including children, adolescents, and pregnant or lactating women. The key is to be aware of your own nutritional needs so that you can plan a diet that meets them.

Vegan diets exclude beef, chicken, and fish, eggs, and dairy products, as well as foods that contain these products. Some people follow a semi-vegetarian diet (also called a flexitarian diet) which is primarily a plant-based diet but includes meat, dairy, eggs, chicken, and fish occasionally or in small amounts. How to plan a healthy vegetarian diet

To get the most out of a vegetarian diet, choose a good variety of healthy plant foods, such as whole fruits and vegetables, legumes, nuts, and whole grains. At the same time, cut down on less healthy options like sugar-sweetened beverages, fruit juices, and refined grains. If you need help, a registered dietitian can help you create a vegetarian plan that is right for you.

To get started

One way to transition to a vegetarian diet is to progressively reduce the meat in your diet while increasing your consumption of fruits and vegetables. Here are a couple of tips to help you get started:

Gradual transition. Increase the number of meatless meals you already enjoy each week, like spaghetti with tomato sauce or stir-fry vegetables. Find ways to include vegetables, such as spinach, kale, chard, and collards, in your daily meals.

Replacements. Take your favorite recipes and try them without meat. For example, make vegetarian chili by omitting the ground beef and adding an extra can of black beans. Or make fajitas using extra firm tofu instead of chicken. You will be surprised to find that many chain rings only require simple replacements.

Diversity. Buy or borrow vegetarian cookbooks. Visit ethnic restaurants to try new vegetarian recipes. The more variety your vegetarian diet has, the more likely you are to meet all of your nutritional needs.

The vegetarian diet, if it is prepared by choosing the foods appropriately and taking into account the guidelines and indications of the doctor or nutritionist, is able to provide the body with the nutrients it needs and to ensure the maintenance of a good state of health.

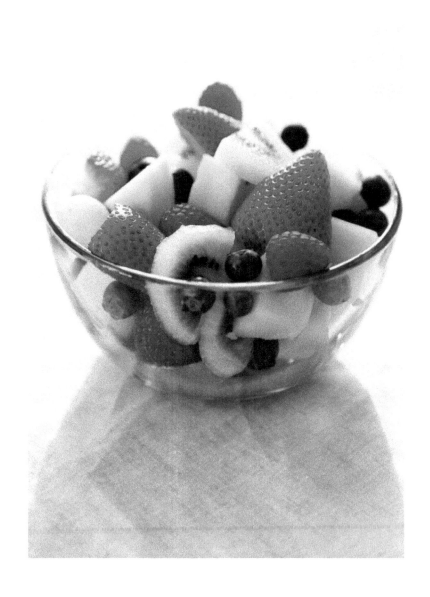